Learner Stronger Energy

Unlock Your Female Fitness Potential and Transform Your Body with Science-Backed from age 20 and above

Rosendo A. Price

Acknowledgment

This book, "Learner Stronger Energy," has been a journey of inspiration, development, and thankfulness. I owe a great deal to the amazing people whose knowledge and insight have influenced how I see the subjects covered in these pages. First and foremost, I would want to express my sincere gratitude to Michael Matthews, whose groundbreaking work in the field of fitness and wellbeing has served as a continual source of inspiration and direction. Your commitment to helping others live their best lives has really motivated me to start this writing and knowledge-sharing journey. I am also very appreciative to [name of another significant author], whose ground-breaking studies and creative concepts have improved my comprehension

Learner Stronger energy

of the fundamentals of energy management and holistic wellbeing. It is a privilege to stand on the shoulders of such giants as you, and your contributions to the field have been essential. I will always be indebted to my family, whose unfailing support and encouragement have been the cornerstone of my success. Through all of this endeavour's highs and lows, your love, tolerance, and understanding have kept me going, and for that, I am very thankful. I am very grateful to my friends and colleagues whose support and criticism helped to develop this book into its final form. Your opinions and thoughts have been priceless, and I am appreciative of the chance to develop along with everyone of you. Lastly, I would like to express my sincere gratitude to all of the readers of this book for their

Learner Stronger energy

support and attention. I really hope that the concepts and viewpoints presented in these pages will encourage you to embrace your own path of personal development, empowerment, and self-discovery. With

Appreciation and modesty,

Rosendo A. Price

CONTENT

Introduction..7

Chapter 1...12

Ignite Your Inner Fire...12

    Unleashing Your Potential..17

    Harnessing Your Mindset for Success.....................22

    Tapping into Your Inner Drive....................................26

Chapter 2...31

    Fuel Your Body, Fuel Your Power.............................31

    Nutrition for Optimal Performance............................35

    Power Foods for Energy and Strength.....................40

    Creating a Sustainable Eating Plan.........................45

Chapter 3...50

    Power Up Your Workouts...50

    Strength Training Essentials.....................................55

    Building Lean Muscle Mass......................................60

    Maximising Your Workout Efficiency.........................67

Chapter 4:..73

    Mind Over Matter: Mental Resilience.......................73

    Overcoming Obstacles and Challenges...................78

    Cultivating Mental Toughness...................................84

    Strategies for Overcoming Plateaus........................89

Chapter 5...96

    Harnessing Your Energy for Life...............................96

    Balancing Fitness and Well-being...........................104

    Integrating Fitness into Your Lifestyle....................112

    Sustaining Your Energy for Long-term Success...121

Conclusion...133

Introduction

The general design of life uncovers a huge reality: Instead of being merely a goal, the path to wellness is a wonderful journey, a huge experience of self-discovery, improvement, and strengthening. Dear reader, welcome to a once-in-a-lifetime adventure that will ignite your passion, awaken your soul, and transform your life in unexpected ways. This is not your typical book; it's an assertion, a manual, a kind of favoured booka a reference point among the chaos and clatter of the remainder of the world. This is your invitation to investigate women's fitness and well-being

Learner Stronger energy

in depth, embark on a journey of self-discovery, and emerge shining, powerful, and unstoppable. You will find the reactions to figuring out your greatest limit, conveying the unlimited energy that is inside you, and building an energetic, strong, and critical life in the pages that follow. From the essentials of activity and diet to the zeniths of mental strength and profound dependability, the parts of this book cover everything. You can consider it a manual to assist you with turning into your best self. However, it cannot be denied that this is not a trip for the weak of heart. It requires fortitude, devotion, and status to go up against one's own evil spirits. It expects you to confront your interests, venture outside your usual comfort zone, and embrace the unknown. In any case, therefore, you will find a wellspring of power that will push you forward as you continue looking for significance—aa strength and versatility you had no clue you had. What can you confidently expect to find within these pages? Be prepared to be awestruck as you read; the wealth that appears to be quite numerous is actually a change. You will sort out some way to get your inward fire going, grasp your unimaginable potential, and encourage a flood and credibility-arranged disposition. You will track down how to deal with your body with food sources that support your spirit, incorporate practice into your standard everyday presence easily and classily, and stay aware of your energy for long-term accomplishment and fulfilment. But the most important thing you'll learn is that your life can be completely changed. You are in charge of your destiny, the primary model for your predetermination, and your ship. Nothing can stop you from achieving your goals because you have the inner fortitude, resiliency, and resolve to conquer whatever stands in your way. Recognise that you have company on this path. You are a member of a group of strong, brave women who support and encourage you at every turn. We will rise, we will prosper, and together, we will build a society where every woman has the ability to live her life to the fullest. So, are you prepared to go off on this amazing journey, my reader? Are you prepared to seize your own opportunities, accept your strength, and design an endlessly happy and fulfilled life? If yes, let's get started. There are an infinite number of options ahead on this voyage. Greetings from a world of boundless possibilities. Greetings on this once-in-a-lifetime excursion. This is your road map to greatness, not simply a book. Let's make each second matter.

Chapter 1

Ignite Your Inner Fire

Imagine a lady asserting her authority and exuding strength, energy, and confidence. What keeps her hidden? It takes more than simply going to the gym and sticking to a strict diet. It's about her inner fire, something deeper and more natural.

"Ignite Your Inner Fire" isn't simply a clever catchphrase. It's an exhortation to women to realise their boundless potential—both intellectually and physically. It's about rekindling the inner flame that gives you motivation, aspiration, and a lifelong love.

Learner Stronger energy

For women, being physically active is about more than simply looking good—it's about feeling strong, powerful, and empowered in all facets of life. It's about taking back control of your health, wellbeing, and physical appearance on your terms.

So, how can you kindle a passion inside yourself for women's fitness?

It all begins, first and foremost, with the mentality. It involves changing your viewpoint from one of opportunity to one of restriction. Pay attention to what you can accomplish rather than what you cannot. Approach your fitness path with joy and curiosity, and accept difficulties as chances for personal development.

The next step is to discover your purpose. What inspires you to exercise each day? Is it the need to feel powerful and secure in your own flesh? Is it the excitement of testing your boundaries and realising your potential? Whatever it is, cling to it firmly since it is what will sustain you in difficult times.

But it takes more than just a positive outlook to kindle your inner fire; you also need to take concrete action. It's about engaging in pursuits that make you feel good on the inside. Perhaps it's the power surge you get from lifting weights with each repetition. Perhaps it's dancing as if no one else is there and enjoying your freedom of movement. Perhaps it's running on trails and experiencing the sensation of the ground under your feet.

Find the thing that lights your soul on fire and give it all you have. Never be afraid to take risks, go outside of your comfort zone, and push yourself to limits you never would have imagined.

And never forget that stoking your inner fire is a continuous activity rather than a one-time occurrence. It's about taking persistent action, taking care of yourself, and loving yourself on a daily basis to fuel that flame. It's about realising that all the time, work, and energy you put into yourself is worthwhile.

The moment is here for all the ladies out there who are prepared to kindle their inner desire to become healthy. Accept the path, accept the difficulty, and accept the woman you were destined to be. Are you prepared to let your inner fire to blaze brightly? It is waiting for you.

Unleashing Your Potential

Every woman possesses a wealth of untapped potential that is just waiting to be unleashed. She possesses a hidden ability that has lain dormant within her, awaiting the appropriate occasion to manifest and alter her life. This potential is not just about having physical strength or athletic brilliance; rather, it is about discovering one's deepest recesses and realising one's true potential.

For women, fitness means more than just maintaining a certain weight or having the ideal figure. The objective is to help them realise their full mental, emotional, and physical potential. Tolerating the vast majority likely lies inside and assuming responsibility for oneself.

However, it's not always easy to reach your full potential. To step outside of your comfort zone requires courage, tenacity, and determination. It involves tolerating disappointment as a vital stage towards accomplishment, standing up to your interests head-on, and never making due with anything short of your absolute best.

All in all, how might you arrive at your maximum capacity regarding female wellness?

Learner Stronger energy

Faith in oneself is the first step. To face any challenge, including your strength and perseverance, you must have faith in your own capabilities. You must have confidence that your true capacity is boundless and that you can accomplish significance.

The subsequent stage is to set bold targets and seek after them with steadfast purpose. Dream enormously and set your sights high, unafraid. Whether it's learning a new yoga pose, finishing a marathon, or deadlifting twice your bodyweight, set goals that push you and inspire you to reach your full potential.

Learner Stronger energy

However, realising your potential requires more than just a regimen of exercise; it also involves your public image. It's tied in with fostering a versatile and development-situated mindset and considering the inability to be an opportunity to get to the next level. It's tied in with putting self-esteem and taking care of oneself first and seeing that caring for yourself isn't self-centred; rather, arriving at your most prominent potential is essential.

It also involves surrounding oneself with positive people who support and believe in one's ability to succeed. Find a gathering of ladies who share your convictions so they can energise, motivate, and support you when you most need it. Both of you can accomplish more than you would have envisioned at any point.

Harnessing Your Mindset for Success

The force of the brain is, in many cases, underestimated in the domain of ladies' wellness. However, our success in life and in the gym ultimately depends on how we think. There's something else involving your attitude for progress besides basically perception practices or hopeful reasoning. It requires cultivating a self-belief mentality that is resilient, tenacious, and persistent.

So, how can you make the most of your thinking to get fit as a woman?

The majority of it involves cultivating a development mindset. Consider issues as any open doors for learning and progress as opposed to as hindrances to survival. Acknowledge disappointment as an important part of the interaction and transform it into inspiration to accomplish. Review that disappointments are simply knocked out and about towards progress; they cannot be overcome.

Rethinking your fitness beliefs and concepts is the next step. Consider how far you've gone and what you can do as opposed to what you can't do or how far you actually need to go. Positive confirmations ought to replace negative self-talk, and you ought to continually help yourself to remember your true capacity, power, and grit.

However, adopting a successful mindset requires more than just optimistic thinking; it also requires consistent action to achieve your goals. Create a plan for achieving your objectives, and set yourself specific, attainable goals. To draw nearer to your prosperity vision, separate your targets into possible stages and earnestly promise to take small, steady exercises.

Understanding that it requires surrounding oneself with positive, upbeat women who share your values is essential. Find a workout partner, join a fitness class, or look for online groups to connect with others who share your goals and ideals. You can encourage one another through trying times, congratulate one another on your accomplishments, and hold one another accountable for your actions together.

Tapping into Your Inner Drive

Every woman has a hidden supply of fortitude, tenacity, and motivation that keeps her moving ahead despite obstacles. Leveraging this innate motivation is essential to realising your whole potential in physical fitness and exercise, enabling you to surpass your boundaries and persistently pursue your objectives.

However, what is this inner drive precisely, and how may one access it?

Your inner drive is fundamentally the fire that burns within you, igniting your enthusiasm for physical fitness and inspiring you to go on through difficult times. It's the inner voice that tells you, "You can do this," when uncertainty starts to seep in. Your gut instinct is what gets you out of bed in the morning, ready to take on your exercise and make the most of the day.

Reaching out to your innermost goals and objectives is the first step towards unleashing your inner drive. What really gets you excited? Regarding what do you have a strong passion for? Find what motivates you and cling to it, whether it's finishing a marathon, learning a new yoga posture, or just feeling strong and secure in your own flesh.

Setting significant objectives that are in line with your inner drive comes next. Your objectives should push you beyond your comfort zone and motivate you to keep going while remaining realistic and difficult. Make a strategy to accomplish each of your objectives one at a time by breaking them down into more manageable, achievable tasks.

In any case, fostering the discretion and backbone to seek after your targets with constancy is just about as significant as having objectives with regards to finding your internal drive. Putting yourself first every day, even when you don't feel like it,

Learner Stronger energy

is the first step. It involves beating agony, vulnerability, and tension with the information that achievement anticipates on the other side.

It's tied in with drawing motivation from the genuine excursion—from the sweat, the difficulty, and the triumphs experienced along the course. Recognise your accomplishments, accept the process, and have faith in your ability to overcome obstacles.

Ladies who are prepared to embrace their inner motivation for physical health and exercise know that they have strength within them. Lay out significant targets,

Learner Stronger energy

foster versatility and poise, interface with your deepest yearnings, and draw motivation from the excursion. When you follow your inner desire, there are no limits to what you can accomplish.

Chapter 2

Fuel Your Body, Fuel Your Power

Your body is an exquisitely balanced apparatus that can do amazing feats of vigour, power, and endurance. To run optimally, however, it needs the proper fuel, just like any other machine. The phrase "Fuel Your Body, Fuel Your Power" serves as a helpful reminder that eating the correct meals can help us reach our maximum potential in terms of fitness and other areas of life.

It takes more than simply monitoring calories or adhering to the newest diet fads to feed your body for strength. It's about giving your body the nourishment it needs to flourish and function at its best—that is, feeding oneself from the inside out.

What does it mean, therefore, to feed your body in order to gain power?

Above all, it's about giving your body the vital vitamins, minerals, and macronutrients it needs to perform at its best—nutrient-dense, whole meals. Think about meals that will promote your general health and well-being in addition to supplying energy for your exercises, such as complex carbs, lean proteins, and healthy fats.

Learner Stronger energy

However, eating the right food is just one aspect of supplying your body with energy; another is eating habits. It involves paying attention to your body's signals of hunger and fullness, eating with awareness, and savouring every mouthful. It's all about striking a balance between treating yourself sometimes and giving priority to nutrient-dense meals that will help you reach your objectives.

The next step is to plan your meals and snacks to maximise your energy levels all day. Before your exercise, fuel yourself with a well-balanced breakfast or snack to help you push through the sweat, and following, refuel to boost muscle repair and refill your energy resources.

The most crucial aspect of fuelling your body for strength, however, may be developing a healthy and empowered connection with food. It involves eschewing diet culture and adopting intuitive eating, which involves paying attention to your body's signs, believing your signals of hunger and fullness, and satisfying your urges without feeling guilty or ashamed.

Nutrition for Optimal Performance

Any effective fitness journey starts with proper nutrition, which gives your body the fundamental building blocks it needs to function at its peak. However, not all meals are made equal when it comes to optimise your performance and feeding your exercises. This is where "Nutrition for Optimal Performance" comes in—a comprehensive eating plan that feeds your body, powers through your exercises, and assists you in reaching your fitness objectives with force and accuracy.

What does nutrition for women's fitness specifically look like for best performance?

The first step is to make nutrient-dense, nutritious meals your top priority. These will provide your body with the energy it needs to fuel your exercises and recover from them. Consider consuming lean proteins to aid in the development and repair of muscles, complex carbs to power your exercise, and healthy fats to maintain hormone balance and provide long-lasting energy.

However, macronutrients alone aren't the only components of proper nutrition; micronutrients, or those vital vitamins and minerals, are also important for general health and wellbeing. Eat a diet rich in fruits and vegetables to provide your body with the vitamins, minerals, and antioxidants it needs to be healthy.

The next step is to plan your meals and snacks to maximise your energy levels all day. Before your activity, feed your body with a balanced meal or snack that includes a mix of protein, carbs, and healthy fats to help minimise tiredness. After your workout, refill your energy reserves and assist muscle recovery.

The most vital part of nourishment for maximised operation, in any case, might be sorting out what your body and you answer best. Find the meal and timing strategy that

Learner Stronger energy

makes you feel full and energised by experimenting. By paying attention to your body's signals of hunger and fullness, you can give in to your urges without feeling guilty or restricted.

Furthermore, always remember that advancement, not flawlessness, is what's genuinely going on with sustenance for maximised operation. Acknowledge adaptability and equilibrium in your eating examples, and focus on furnishing your body with sustenance from feasts that support your certainty and provide you with a feeling of solidarity.

Learner Stronger energy

The power is presently in your grasp, women who are ready to improve their presentations and fuel their activities. Make whole, nutrient-rich meals your top priority. Eat with mindfulness. Focus on your body's signs. By giving your body the right supplements, you'll fuel your activities as well as give yourself the strength and certainty you need to reach your wellness goals.

Power Foods for Energy and Strength

The right eating routine might significantly affect ladies' wellness and exercise execution by expanding energy levels, advancing solid turns of events, and working on broad wellbeing. These are what we call "power foods," which are tasty and high in nutrients that give your body the energy it needs to smash your fitness goals and take control of your workouts.

So, what exactly are power meals, and how might they benefit women's fitness?

Learner Stronger energy

Macronutrients, which are the proteins, lipids, and carbohydrates that make up strength and energy, make up the majority of power meals. Your body involves sugars as a fast-consuming fuel for serious activity; proteins help in the turn of events and fix of muscles; and solid fats keep up with chemical equilibrium while providing durable energy.

Power food varieties high in carbs incorporate organic products like bananas and berries, nutritious grains like earthy-coloured rice and quinoa, and boring vegetables like butternut squash and yams. These feasts give your body a predictable stockpile of energy to assist you with even the most demanding exercise.

For women's fitness, lean protein foods like turkey, tofu, lentils, fish, and poultry are excellent choices. By giving your muscles the fundamental amino acids they need to become more grounded and mend after an exercise, these feasts will assist you with acquiring fit bulk and accelerate your metabolism in the middle of meetings.

omitting the significance of healthy fats. Avocado, nuts, seeds, and olive oil are good fats that help make hormones and give you energy for a long time. In addition to improving your overall health and wellbeing, including these foods in your diet will help you feel full and energised throughout the day.

However, macronutrients aren't the only components of power meals; they also include a wealth of micronutrients, including vitamins, minerals, and antioxidants, which promote optimum performance and recovery. For women's health and activity, colourful veggies like bell peppers and carrots, antioxidant-rich fruits like oranges and kiwis, and leafy greens like spinach and kale are all great options.

Learner Stronger energy

The options are thus unlimited for all the ladies out there who are prepared to give their bodies power meals to give them strength and vitality. To identify what works best for you, try a range of nutrient-rich meals, taste and texture combinations, and pay attention to your body's signals. You may improve your general health and vitality, as well as your energy and strength, by feeding your body the correct meals.

Creating a Sustainable Eating Plan

When it comes to achieving your fitness goals, what you eat and how you exercise are just as important as one another. In any case, with so many eating regimens and famous styles and examples accessible, it may very well be hard to tell where to start. Thus, making a feasible eating plan is urgent—a delectable and special methodology that upholds actual work, long-term wellbeing, and yearning fulfilment.

So, for women's health and well-being, what exactly does it mean to create an affordable eating plan?

The most urgent thing to remember is to track down balance. A sustainable eating plan places less emphasis on starvation or restriction and more on eating a wide variety of foods in moderation and paying attention to your body's signals of hunger and fullness. The mystery is to pick dinners that will fuel your body and satisfy your cravings without settling on taste or satisfaction.

The next stage is to focus on eating entire, supplement-rich dinners that give your body the crucial macronutrients, nutrients, and minerals it needs to flourish. Not only will eating meals that are high in whole grains, lean proteins, and healthy fats help you exercise, but they will also improve your overall health and wellbeing.

But merely altering your diet isn't enough to create a sustainable eating plan; it also requires dietary adjustments. It involves eating carefully, appreciating each significant chomp, and focusing on your body's general longing and satisfaction signals. It is more important to enjoy eating than to rush through meals or nibble incessantly.

The ability to adapt is the next topic. A budget diet plan prioritises progress over perfection. During the cycle, you should adjust as necessary to find what works best for you and your body. It has to do with permitting yourself to intermittently partake in your most noteworthy hits without feeling remorseful or embarrassed.

The issue of sustainability comes up last. If an eating plan helps you reach your goals and fits your lifestyle without putting you under too much stress or restriction, you might stick with it for the long haul. Finding a daily schedule of eating sustains your body, fulfils your cravings, and urges you to work out.

In this way, ladies, the power is presently in your grasp in the event that you're prepared

Learner Stronger energy

to make an enduring eating regimen plan for wellness. Eat mindfully, embrace change, and place sustainability at the top of your priority list to achieve equilibrium. You can support your workout routine and improve your overall health and wellbeing for many years to come by providing your body with delicious and nutritious food.

Chapter 3

Power Up Your Workouts

What does it truly intend to "power up" your activities, then, at that point?

The most important thing is to create the conditions for success. Start by giving your body the right nutrients to ensure that you have the stamina and energy to push through your workouts. To take care of your muscles and advance your greatest execution, pick supplement-rich, complete feasts that incorporate an equilibrium of carbs, proteins, and solid fats.

The next step is to determine the ideal intensity-to-recovery ratio. Listen to your body, give yourself the rest and recuperation you need, and push yourself to new heights and overcome obstacles to avoid burnout and injury. To keep your body interested and your progress moving forward, combine vigorous exercise with active recuperation days.

However, in order to get the most out of your workouts, being mentally prepared is just as important as being physically prepared. Set specific goals for each exercise, and imagine yourself easily achieving them. Create a positive and inspiring mentality that serves as a constant reminder of your strength, resilience, and capacity to overcome obstacles.

The next stage is to adjust your structure and strategy to obtain the most ideal results while staying away from harm. In every activity you engage in, give proper form and alignment top priority, and prioritise quality over quantity. Consider working with a certified personal trainer or fitness coach to ensure that each exercise is performed safely and effectively.

Last but not least, it's all about having fun and getting excited about working out.

Learner Stronger energy

Introduce new workouts, courses, or formats to keep things interesting and prevent boredom. Choose activities like weightlifting, yoga, or dancing to your favourite music that you really enjoy and that give you a sense of power and vitality.

The second is hanging around for every one of the women out there who are ready to move forward with their activities and arrive at their most noteworthy location, likely the exercise centre. Keep a solid eating regimen, find some kind of harmony among effort and recovery, centre around the right structure, have a great time all through your exercises, and make a decent standpoint. You'll be amazed at what you can do in the rec centre and beyond it, assuming you take the legitimate disposition.

Strength Training Essentials

A key component of a successful strategy for achieving your fitness goals is strength training. However, for many women, the idea of lifting weights may be unsettling or apprehensive. Knowing the fundamentals of strength training is, therefore, essential. In the gym, you can use this tasty and unique method to build resilience, strength, and confidence.

Therefore, what specific components of strength training are required for women's fitness?

Recognising the benefits of strength training and how it can alter your life and body is essential. As well as expanding strength and solid mass, strength preparation likewise advances temperament, increments digestion, works on bone thickness, and brings down the opportunity of injury. A successful technique for fostering a physical make-up serious areas of strength for is being confident from the back to the front.

The next step is to master the fundamental movements that support any strength training program. Compound activities that focus on various strong gatherings and give the most bang to your cash include squats, deadlifts, jumps, presses, and lines. Start with bodyweight versions of these exercises to build a solid foundation, then progress to using weights as you get stronger.

However, knowledge of important concepts like increasing overload, proper form, and recuperation is included in the fundamentals of strength training in addition to the exercises themselves. With the end goal of ceaselessly pushing your muscles and empowering improvement, moderate overburden alludes to logically expanding the weight, reiterations, or sets of your exercises after some time. Prior to adding weight, work on perfecting your form, which is essential for maximising performance and avoiding injuries. Also, keep in mind the significance of recovery. To forestall overtraining and burnout, make certain to allow your muscles time to recuperate and loosen in the middle of workouts.

Finding a strength training programme that suits your needs and way of life is the next step. There are several ways to include strength training in your routine, whether you like to lift weights at the gym, follow along with online programmes at home, or enrol in a group fitness class. Try out a variety of formats and techniques to see what suits you best, and don't be scared to switch things up to make your exercises engaging and difficult.

Ultimately, it's about appreciating your progress along the road and accepting the ride. Every exercise is a chance to challenge yourself, become stronger, and become the greatest version of yourself. Strength training is a path of self-discovery and empowerment. The world is yours to conquer, so lace up your trainers, grab some weights, and get ready to release your inner power.

Building Lean Muscle Mass

Acquiring fit bulk is an extraordinary encounter that includes creating flexibility, strength, and certainty from the back to the front. It goes beyond working on one's actual look. Even though women may be hesitant or apprehensive about the idea, building lean muscle mass is really one of the most powerful things you can do for your body and health.

Building lean muscle is more than just looking good. It's about being useful and living a good life. As well as adding structure and definition to your body, slender bulk raises energy levels, advances

Learner Stronger energy

general wellbeing and prosperity, increments digestion, and works on bone thickness. It's a useful tool that can help you feel strong, confident, and capable in many areas of your life.

All in all, how unequivocally does a woman approach acquiring slender bulk?

The bulk of it deals with resistance training. Lean solid mass might be assembled and muscle improvement invigorated most really by strength preparation with loads or obstruction groups. Focus on complex developments like squats, deadlifts, thrusts, presses, and columns that work numerous strong gatherings at the same time. To keep your muscles challenged and encouraged to improve, gradually increase the resistance while working with lighter weights as you gain strength.

Nonetheless, acquiring slender bulk requires more than essentially lifting loads; you additionally need to take care of your body in the right way to advance both muscle improvement and recuperation. give need to feasts high in protein, like poultry, turkey, fish, tofu, and lentils. Your muscles get the essential amino acids they need to grow and heal from these foods. To give your body the energy and nutrition it needs to build muscle and power through your exercises, combine your protein with healthy fats like avocado, nuts, seeds, and olive oil, also l as complex carbohydrates like whole grains, fruits, and vegetables.

Next, consistency and progress are essential. Keep up with your diet and exercise routine, because building lean muscle mass takes time and effort. At the very least, try to do strength training three to four times per week. To continue pushing your muscles and empowering advancement, dynamically increase the volume and force of your activities. To keep yourself responsible and propelled on your way, measure, take pictures, or record your solidarity increments consistently.

Developing a mentality is possibly the most crucial aspect of gaining lean muscle development. It all comes down to having confidence in your own abilities to reach your objectives, especially in the face of obstacles or sluggish progress. Develop an optimistic and self-empowering perspective that celebrates your accomplishments along the journey and serves as a constant reminder of your strength, resiliency, and potential. Recall that gaining lean muscle mass is a journey rather than a goal, so enjoy the experience and have faith in your body's capacity to change and become stronger with each training session.

Thus, the moment has come for all ladies who are eager to develop lean muscle mass and discover their inner power. Adopt a resistance training regimen, eat healthily, exercise consistently and progressively, and have a positive outlook that will enable you to reach your full potential. You can change your body and your life from the inside out by gaining lean muscle mass with commitment, perseverance, and a little bit of sweat.

Learner Stronger energy

Maximising Your Workout Efficiency

Making the most of your gym time and obtaining the best outcomes with the least amount of effort is the key to maximising the effectiveness of your workouts. Since time is of the essence for women, it's critical to maximise every minute of your exercises. The following are some crucial tactics to improve the effectiveness of your workouts:

Plan Ahead: Spend some time organising your exercise before you ever enter the gym. Choose the exercises you'll complete, the number of sets and repetitions you'll do, and the amount of time you'll rest in between sets. Making the most of your time and maintaining concentration may be achieved by having a well-defined strategy in place.

Concentrate on Compound Movements: Compound movements are your greatest buddy when it comes to optimising exercise efficiency. These workouts, which include squats, deadlifts, lunges, presses, and rows, target many muscular groups simultaneously. You may target numerous muscles in one workout and get more value for your money by concentrating on compound motions.

Employ Supersets and Circuits: By cutting down on the amount of time you spend resting between exercises, supersets and circuits are two advanced training strategies that may help you get the most out of your workouts. Targeting distinct muscle groups, a superset consists of doing two exercises back-to-back without a break in between. During a circuit, you do a set of exercises one after the other with little to no break in between. Your exercises will be more effective if you can do more work in less time using these approaches.

Limit Rest Periods: Taking excessively lengthy breaks in between sets is one of the greatest time wasters in the gym. Even while recovery requires rest, brief rest intervals may help you sustain intensity and raise your heart rate throughout the exercise. Try to maximise the amount of time you spend resting between sets by limiting it to 60–90 seconds.

Make High-Intensity Intervals a Priority: HIIT training is another efficient strategy to increase exercise efficiency. Short bursts of high-intensity activity are interspersed with rest or lower-intensity exercise during high-intensity interval training (HIIT). This increases metabolism and strengthens your cardiovascular system in addition to

Learner Stronger energy

assisting you in burning more calories in less time.

While pushing yourself throughout your exercises is crucial, it's as important to pay attention to your body and know when to back off. Give yourself enough time to relax and recuperate in between sessions to avoid burnout and injury from overtraining. Do not be afraid to take a day off or choose a less intense exercise if you are feeling exhausted or exhausted.

Also to optimum effectiveness and performance, remember to keep hydrated and fed during your exercise. Stay hydrated

Learner Stronger energy

by drinking plenty of water prior to, during, and after your exercise. To promote muscle repair and energy production, feed your body with a balanced meal or snack that includes protein, carbs, and healthy fats.

You may increase the effectiveness of your workouts and get the best results faster by putting these techniques into practice. This will free up more time for you to enjoy the activities you like outside of the gym.

Chapter 4:

Mind Over Matter: Mental Resilience

With regards to wellbeing and wellness, mental sturdiness is in many cases the unrecognised yet truly great individual that drives long-term achievement and actual change. It is the capacity to overcome obstacles, persevere through difficulties, and remain focused on your goals. Moreover, creating mental strength is fundamental for ladies to flourish in all aspects of life and to meet their wellness targets.

Learner Stronger energy

What exactly is mental resilience, and how can women cultivate this strong mentality?

Mental versatility is generally a disposition. It's about adopting a positive and powerful perspective that enables you to persevere and gracefully deal with life's ups and downs. It involves altering your perspective on failures as opportunities for personal growth, accepting challenges as opportunities for improvement, and having faith in your own capacity to overcome any obstacle.

Notwithstanding, mental strength likewise includes mindfulness, which is the capacity to recognise and control your considerations, sentiments, and ways of behaving in a way that advances your prosperity. Managing stress, being aware of your stresses and triggers, and asking for help from friends, family, or experts when necessary are all part of this.

Next, perseverance is the key to mental resilience; it is tied in with sticking to your goals and proceeding to act reliably even despite difficulty. It's about setting reasonable expectations, breaking down big goals into smaller, more manageable tasks, and appreciating your progress. Accepting the journey and having faith in your ability to achieve your goals, no matter how long it takes or how many obstacles you face, are the keys to success.

Perhaps most importantly, however, mental resilience is just about resilience: it's about rising stronger and more determined than ever after experiencing disappointment, rejection, or failure. It's about seeing obstacles as chances for development and education instead of as indicators of inadequacy or failure. It's about picking yourself up, getting back up on your feet, and entering the game with fresh concentration and resolve.

Thus, the moment has come for all the ladies out there who are prepared to develop mental toughness and realise their full potential. Adopt a constructive and empowering outlook, engage in self-awareness and self-care, endure hardships, and overcome failures with more vigour than before. You may flourish in all facets of life and realise your aspirations of living the life you've always wanted by developing mental resilience. This will help you reach your fitness objectives.

Overcoming Obstacles and Challenges

The road to health and fitness is not without its challenges. When it comes to achieving their fitness goals, women frequently face a number of challenges, including a lack of time, money, motivation, or injuries or plateaus. However, it is doable to overcome these challenges and emerge stronger, healthier, and more self-assured than before.

Above all else, it's basic to perceive that hardships and road obstructions are an inescapable part of the journey for wellbeing and prosperity. Instead of seeing them as obstacles or disappointments, see them as opportunities for growth and education. You might change your perspective and defy hindrances with certainty and resolve by outlining them as any open doors to becoming more grounded and stronger.

The next significant step is to recognise and appreciate the specific obstructions and troubles you are experiencing. Do you struggle to find time to exercise on a regular basis? Is it difficult for you to remain motivated to finish your exercises? Or then again, perhaps you're apprehensive about falling flat, which keeps you from venturing beyond your usual range of familiarity. By determining the root causes of your issues, you can focus your strategies on overcoming obstacles and moving towards your goals.

A useful strategy for overcoming difficulties is to break them down into smaller, more manageable phases. Think about each issue or obstacle in turn and make a game plan to settle it, as opposed to endeavouring to deal with everything simultaneously. It can be more manageable and less overwhelming to break down large tasks into smaller steps. Finding an accountability partner or workout buddy to keep you motivated, setting realistic goals, and acknowledging your progress along the way are all examples of this. Other examples of this include planning your workouts ahead of time to make time for them.

Another important strategy for overcoming obstacles is to ask for help and advice from others. Gathering an organisation of individuals who put stock in you and your objectives, whether it be through employing a fitness coach, joining a wellness local area or care group, or asking companions or family who have gone through comparative battles for direction,

Learner Stronger energy

can be a gigantic wellspring of motivation and support on your excursion.

Last but not least, it's essential to remember that difficulties and setbacks are unavoidable and do not signify failure. Rather than permitting disappointments to debilitate you or hinder your progress, consider them to be opportunities for self-improvement and schooling. Recollect the illustrations you gained from the occasion, change your system on a case-by-case basis, and continue with new diligence and determination.

You are in good company with women who are experiencing challenges and boundaries in their quest for wellness. You can overcome any test and arrive at your wellness targets with the assistance of others, a decent standpoint, centred procedures, and a longing to learn and create. You'll be prepared to live the bright, healthy life you deserve once you do these things.

Cultivating Mental Toughness

Mental strength is a strong expertise that can change how you approach wellness and enable you to beat obstructions, continue on through difficulties, and arrive at your objectives. Building mental sturdiness in women incorporates making genuine strength as well as inner power and sureness to overcome deterrents while heading to prosperity.

The most important move towards creating mental strength is developing a disposition of versatility that empowers you to get through difficulty. It's about adopting a positive attitude and viewing setbacks as learning opportunities rather than impediments that cannot be overcome. By adjusting your point of view and tolerating mishaps as any open doors for development and accomplishment, you can foster the strength and persistence important to conquer any hindrance.

The subsequent stage in further developing mental strength is to set clear, achievable objectives and stick to them in any event, even when circumstances become difficult. It all comes down to figuring out what your fitness goals are and breaking them down into smaller, more manageable chunks that you can focus on every day. Despite obstacles or failures, setting savvy (explicit, quantifiable, feasible, significant, and time-bound) goals can help you stay focused and convinced.

Developing a resilient attitude is just as important as learning coping mechanisms for stressful situations, overcoming obstacles, and maintaining motivation. When things get too much, it's important to practice self-care and stress reduction techniques like yoga, meditation, or deep breathing. It's about learning positive ways to deal with problems, like writing, talking to friends, or taking up a favourite hobby, which will help you get back up and see things from a new angle. It also requires you to locate sources of motivation and inspiration that motivate you to persevere through difficult times.

There are two successful techniques for creating mental courage: putting yourself in a position where you have to step outside of your comfort zone on a regular basis and allowing yourself to feel pain. Mental toughness, resilience, and self-assurance may develop when you push yourself to lift heavier weights, try a new programme, or increase the intensity of your training. You can foster more prominent versatility, strength, and confidence that you are fit for beating any deterrent by tolerating distress and driving yourself to change and develop.

In the end, the only way to improve mental toughness is to acknowledge one's progress and accomplishments. Recognising your progress and rewarding yourself for your diligence and effort are at the heart of this. At the point when you recognise and value your achievements, regardless of how little they might be, you will feel more persuaded and certain. Your self-belief and ability to achieve your goals will be bolstered by this.

As a result, women all over the world now have the chance to alter their health habits and cultivate mental toughness. To cultivate a resilient mindset, establish specific goals, develop coping strategies, acknowledge discomfort, and celebrate successes as you go. If you are steadfast, committed, and prepared to go beyond your comfort zone, you can develop the mental fortitude necessary to overcome obstacles and achieve your health objectives. Through this, you can develop into your most grounded and best self.

Strategies for Overcoming Plateaus

A typical obstacle that many women encounter while pursuing fitness is plateauing. Stumbling upon a plateau, whether it related to weight reduction, strength training, or advancement, may be disheartening and distressing. But have no fear—there are techniques you may utilise to get over obstacles and keep pushing with confidence and will towards your fitness objectives.

Priority one should be given to understanding the underlying reasons for plateaus. When your body adjusts to your present training programme and stops responding to the same stimuli, plateaus often develop. This might occur when you do the same exercises repeatedly without change or when you don't push yourself to the limit via progressive overload. You may create focused methods to overcome your plateau and keep moving forward by figuring out what's causing it.

Changing up your exercise regimen is a good way to get past a plateau. This might include adding new exercises, adjusting the intensity or sequence of your sessions, or experimenting with whole alternative training methodologies. You may push your muscles in novel ways and encourage development and adaptation by varying up your exercises. This will help you overcome workout plateaus and keep moving closer to your objectives.

Concentrating on gradual overload is another tactic for getting beyond plateaus. Progressive overload refers to increasing the volume, intensity, or length of your exercises gradually in order to keep pushing your muscles and encouraging development. This might include using larger weights, doing more repetitions or sets, or taking fewer breaks in between workouts. You may break through plateaus and reach new heights of strength and fitness by gradually stressing your muscles to keep them engaged and avoid stagnation.

Being persistent and patient is, however, perhaps one of the most crucial tactics for getting beyond plateaus. In the fitness journey, plateaus are a normal occurrence and frequently signify the body's readiness for a breakthrough. Keep moving ahead with tenacity and commitment, staying focused on your objectives rather than giving up or becoming disheartened. Have faith in the process and trust that you will overcome your plateau and keep moving closer to your objectives with patience and persistence.

It's crucial to pay attention to several elements that might affect your growth, such as diet, sleep, stress, and recuperation, in addition to varying up your training routine and concentrating on progressive overload. In order to support your workouts and recuperation, make sure you're giving your body the nutrition it needs, getting enough sleep and rest to enable your muscles to develop and heal, and controlling your stress levels to avoid tiredness and burnout.

You can overcome plateaus and keep moving towards your fitness objectives by using these techniques and being patient and persistent. This will give you the tools you need to become the healthiest and strongest version of yourself.

Chapter 5

Harnessing Your Energy for Life

Fostering an existence of direction, enthusiasm, and satisfaction is conceivable when you figure out how to saddle your boundless inward energy. Beyond simply maintaining physical vitality, this is a life-altering experience. Women's energy use requires more than just being alert and active; it also involves encouraging vitality and overall health in all aspects of life.

Understanding and regarding your body's intrinsic cycles and necessities is the most vital move towards completely using your energy. It's about listening to your body's signals, allowing yourself to exercise when you're feeling energetic and rest when you're tired, and eating nutritious meals to fuel your body and mind. Through the most common way of tuning into your body's regular insight, you might boost your energy and work on your overall wellbeing and essentialness.

Notwithstanding, utilising your energy includes more than basically keeping up with your actual wellbeing; it additionally involves fostering your otherworldliness, mental clarity, and close-to-home backbone. It includes utilising procedures

Learner Stronger energy

like care, contemplation, and breathwork to loosen up the sensory system and calm the brain so you might get a more significant sensation of present and tranquilly in your everyday exercises. It's about improving your emotional intelligence and self-awareness so that you can deal with life's ups and downs with grace and resilience. Viewing importance and reason in your way likewise includes making an association with an option that could be greater than yourself, whether it is confidence, a local area, or the normal world.

Learner Stronger energy

Making opportunity and energy for pursuits and associations that move and rouse you is an incredible procedure to carry on with a long and solid life. This could be participating in a creative endeavour, spending time outdoors, or strengthening relationships with people you care about. You might refuel your energy reserves and make an obviously brilliant sensation of power and prosperity by encircling yourself with positive energy and taking care of your soul with pursuits that please and charm you.

Schedules and habits that support your mental, spiritual, and actual prosperity should also help you feel more energetic. This could incorporate consistently working on, eating well, getting sufficient rest, and utilising pressure-relieving procedures like yoga or journaling. By prioritising self-care and well-being in your day-to-day activities, you can build a foundation of health and energy that enables you to fully participate in all aspects of your life and perform at your best.

Living a life that is in line with your values, interests, and goals is the most important thing you can do to get the most out of your energy. Identifying your interests and areas of enjoyment and pursuing them with

Learner Stronger energy

enthusiasm and responsibility is essential. Living genuinely gives you access to a perpetual stock of energy and imperativeness that gives your life meaning, whether you decide to seek after a vocation that is in accordance with your qualities, take part in imaginative leisure activities, or reward the local area in significant ways.

As a consequence of this, the time has come for each and every woman who is willing to give their lives to this cause. Spread out strong timetables and inclinations, give need to people and things that give you energy, recognise the body's ordinary cycles, work on mental and significant fortitude, and continue with a day-to-day presence that is consistent with your convictions, interests, and mission. By contributing your energy in these ways, you could maintain a day-to-day presence filled with centrality, fulfilment, and reason. You can also make the most of your life and have a significant impact on your surroundings by putting your energy to use.

This exploration of the idea of harnessing energy for life emphasises the importance of developing mental clarity and emotional resilience, tuning into the body's natural rhythms, prioritising energising activities and relationships, and living in alignment

Learner Stronger energy

with values and purpose in order to achieve

vitality, purpose, and fulfilment in life.

Balancing Fitness and Well-being

In the present high-speed world, numerous ladies should gently adjust their prosperity and wellness. To foster an existence of energy, joy, and satisfaction, it is essential to find harmony between mental prosperity, close-to-home equilibrium, actual wellbeing, and profound arrangement. For ladies, keeping a good arrangement among wellness and prosperity includes more than just looking lovely; it also includes having a decent outlook on themselves and cultivating all-encompassing health in all aspects of life.

Learner Stronger energy

Setting taking care of oneself and self-empathy as a main concern is the most vital move towards finding some kind of harmony among wellbeing and wellness. Acknowledging that caring for your necessities isn't self-centred yet rather fundamental to your general prosperity. This could mean setting aside a few minutes from your rushed schedule for actual work, rest, and satisfying pursuits that renew your body, brain, and soul. If you prioritise self-care and set time and energy limits, wellness may flourish in your life.

Notwithstanding, keeping up with mental and profound health is similarly pretty much as significant as keeping up with actual wellbeing while finding some kind of harmony between wellness and prosperity. To foster a decent viewpoint and profound flexibility even with life's snags, one should rehearse care and mindfulness. It's tied in with understanding when to request help and when to search out associations and backing from companions, family, or specialists when vital. It additionally includes finding helpful ways of dealing with especially difficult times for pressure and overburden, like composition, reflection, or cheerful inventive undertakings.

Learner Stronger energy

A helpful methodology for finding some kind of harmony among wellbeing and wellness is to embrace a comprehensive perspective that considers the connection between the psyche, body, and soul. This could mean adding qigong, yoga, or tai chi to your workout routine to help you build strength, flexibility, and relaxation while also supporting your mental and emotional health. It could likewise incorporate giving main concern to pursuits that inspire and nourish your soul, for example, going on nature strolls, doing local area administration, or integrating care and appreciation into your regular daily schedule.

Learner Stronger energy

Another essential strategy for achieving a healthy balance between fitness and health is to cultivate a positive relationship with food and nutrition. Think of food as food for your body and soul, as opposed to exercise fuel. A decent eating routine brimming with complete, supplement-rich food varieties that help your actual wellbeing and energy levels ought to be your fundamental concentration, yet you ought to likewise here and there enjoy delights and guilty pleasures that make you blissful and fulfilled. Through careful eating that praises your cravings and focuses on your body's signs of yearning and totality, you might

Learner Stronger energy

foster a solid relationship with food and upgrade your general prosperity.

Finding satisfaction and happiness in the process is potentially the most critical part of finding some kind of harmony among wellness and prosperity. It's tied in with valuing the little victories along the way and tolerating the excursion of self-revelation and progress. Find thoroughly enjoying the current second and relishing the wealth of life's encounters, whether it's hitting another wellness objective, having a quiet, clear second during reflection, or simply investing some energy alone in nature. You might foster an unmistakable inclination towards prosperity that exudes from the inside and empowers you to carry on with your best life by embracing a demeanour of gratitude and appreciation for the outing.

The second is here, women, for those of you who are ready to figure out some kind of harmony among wellbeing and wellness. Focus on taking care of oneself and self-sympathy; cultivate all-encompassing prosperity in the body, psyche, and soul; cultivate a positive relationship with nutrition and food; and, what's more, find bliss and happiness en route. By finding a balance between fitness and well-being in these ways, you can design a life that is full of energy, pleasure, and fulfilment, be prepared to live your best life, and positively influence the world around you.

Integrating Fitness into Your Lifestyle

Squeezing practices into your timetable is just one part of coordinating wellness into your way of life; the other is creating a comprehensive health and wellness plan that incorporates regular physical activity into every aspect of your life. Rather than merely achieving a certain body type or size, incorporating fitness for women involves cultivating vitality, energy, and resilience to thrive in all facets of life.

Accepting that movement is normal and necessary is the first step in incorporating exercise into your routine. Consider practice as an opportunity to move your body, support your spirits, and feed your spirit, as opposed to an obligation or errand. This might be finding a great time for regular errands like utilising the steps rather than the lift or doing squats while cleaning your teeth, or it very well may be finding satisfaction in basic distractions like strolling, moving, or planting. You can easily integrate practice into your ordinary daily schedule and develop a lifetime propensity for wellbeing and imperativeness by tolerating development as a blissful articulation of taking care of oneself.

Learner Stronger energy

Nonetheless, keeping up with mental and profound prosperity is basically as significant as expanding actual activity with regards to integrating wellness into your way of life. It's tied in with involving exercise as a viable device to lessen pressure, lift mind-set, and support consideration and mental clarity. Find exercises that challenge your body as well as sustain your psyche and soul. Going for a run to unwind after a long day, doing yoga to find inner peace and balance, or going to the gym to get rid of stress and make more endorphins are examples of such activities. By prioritising your mental and emotional health, you can lead a lifestyle that encourages overall health and vitality.

Making exercise enjoyable and agreeable is one way to integrate it into your day-to-day schedule effectively. Instead of viewing exercise as a solitary pastime, find ways to incorporate it into group outings, trips, and activities. Joining a games group, going to a gathering wellness class, or taking a stroll with companions are only a couple of instances of how turning out with others might expand exercise's feeling of tomfoolery and commitment while likewise offering social help and obligation. You might focus on your wellbeing and prosperity while at the same time strengthening your associations with others by including social and cooperative perspectives into your gym routine and daily practice.

Another important strategy for incorporating exercise into your daily routine is creating a welcoming environment that inspires you to live an active and healthy lifestyle. This could mean setting up a home gym or workout area that is inviting and comfortable, stocking your kitchen with healthy foods that nourish your body and mind, and surrounding yourself with positive role models and people who inspire you to put your health and well-being first. By arranging your environment to support your fitness goals, you can set yourself up for success and make it easier to stay committed to your health journey.

The most essential part of integrating exercise into your daily schedule, nonetheless, might be tracking down an equilibrium and versatility that suit you. It's tied in with focusing on your body's signs and regarding your necessities for both development and movement, as well as rest, recovery, and recharging. It's about taking pleasure in the little victories and achievements you make along the way and treating yourself with kindness and compassion, even when you don't feel like working out. You might plan a way of life that advances your wellbeing and prosperity and accounts for suddenness, delight, and satisfaction by taking on a mentality of equilibrium and adaptability.

In this manner, now is the ideal opportunity for every one of the women out there who are ready to incorporate activity into their regular routines. Acknowledge development as a pleasurable method for rehearsing taking care of oneself; give mental and close-to-home prosperity as

Learner Stronger energy

the as the primary goal; make it fun and social to exercise; create an environment that is supportive; and figure out what kind of balance and adaptability suit you best. You might construct a day-to-day existence that is energetic, upbeat, and satisfying by integrating exercise into your way of life in these ways. This will empower you to prosper in all parts of your life.

To accomplish comprehensive wellbeing and essentialness, this request investigates integrating exercise into your way of life for ladies in a human and important way, featuring the meaning of mindset, social

Learner Stronger energy

help, natural plan, equilibrium, and adaptability.

Sustaining Your Energy for Long-term Success

Accomplishing your goals and carrying on with a fantastic life rely vigorously on keeping up with your energy for long-term achievement. It includes creating schedules and ways of behaving that help your body, psyche, and soul and assist you with supporting your greatest energy and imperativeness over the course of time. Keeping up with energy for ladies includes more than absolutely traversing the day; it additionally includes cultivating versatility and complete prosperity so they might prevail in all aspects of life.

Learner Stronger energy

Prioritising one's own self-care and self-awareness is the most important part of maintaining vitality. Respecting your body's needs for relaxation, hydration, exercise, and renewal requires being aware of your body's cues. This may be taking stops to unwind and re-energise while required, eating a solid eating regimen that will provide your body with energy that will endure over the course of the day, and getting sufficient rest every night to recharge your batteries. It is feasible to lay the groundwork for wellbeing and imperativeness that advances long-term achievement and prosperity by focusing on taking care of oneself and your body's signs.

But keeping your mental and emotional health the same is just as important as keeping your physical health for staying alive. It involves developing habits that promote mental, emotional, and inner peace as well as strategies for reducing stress. This might be journaling to handle feelings and gain knowledge about your viewpoints and sentiments, rehearsing care contemplation to quiet the brain and alleviate stress, or participating in satisfying and happy imaginative undertakings. By placing a high value on your psychological and profound prosperity, you might foster strength and equilibrium that will assist you with overcoming the ups and downs of life.

To keep up with your energy for long-term achievement, foster schedules and ways of behaving that advance your overall prosperity. This may entail incorporating exercise and movement into your daily routine to boost your mood and energy levels, using time management skills to prioritise jobs and activities that align with your values and goals, and creating a morning ritual that makes you feel good about the day ahead. You might foster the energy and consistency important to drive

Learner Stronger energy

yourself towards long-term achievement and bliss by framing schedules and propensities that advance your wellbeing and prosperity.

Another important way to keep your energy up is to create a supportive environment that encourages growth. Keep yourself encompassed by sure and motivating individuals, and search for mentally animating and testing learning that opens doors for yourself. Your motivation and enthusiasm for long-term success can be fueled by investing in your own personal development. A few instances of this incorporate finding coaches and good examples who can give direction and backing, joining a strong local area of similar people, and partaking in proficient improvement exercises that upgrade your abilities and information.

The capacity to strike a balance between your values, interests, and goals is possibly the most important aspect of maintaining your motivation for long-term success. It involves making decisions that honour your authentic self, advance your vision for the future, and lead a life of authenticity and meaning. Expressing no to responsibilities and exercises that sap your energy and remove you from your goals may be one method for doing this, as could expressing yes to chances that fit with your qualities and make you cheerful and satisfied. By living in accordance with your values and purpose, you can maintain your energy and enthusiasm for the long term, be empowered to achieve your goals, and lead a fulfilling and purposeful life.

Subsequently, the second is currently for every one of the women out there who are ready to keep up with their energies for long-haul achievement. Focus on mental and profound wellbeing, foster schedules and propensities that advance your prosperity, encircle yourself with steady

Learner Stronger energy

individuals and settings, focus on taking care of oneself and mindfulness, and live really and deliberately as per your convictions and mission. You might accomplish long-term achievement and joy by keeping up with your energy in these ways, which will empower you to thrive in all aspects of your life.

To make long-term progress and satisfaction, this investigation dives into supporting energy for ladies' drawn-out outcomes in a human and engaging manner, stressing the meaning of taking care of oneself, mental and profound

Learner Stronger energy

health, schedules and propensities, steady conditions, and living truly and deliberately.

Conclusion

This present time is the perfect open door to think about the persevering effect of the data allowed in these pages as we approach the end of our excursion together. All through this book, we have dove profoundly into ladies' wellness and prosperity, uncovering influential ideas, methodologies, and practices to help you while heading to imperativeness, strength, and happiness.

Each section has been filled in as a declaration of your groundbreaking potential, whether it be to stoke your inner fire, build mental fortitude, incorporate

Learner Stronger energy

wellness into your lifestyle, or maintain your motivation for long-term success. You have acknowledged the possibility that genuine wellbeing incorporates mental, close-to-home, and profound prosperity, notwithstanding actual wellbeing. You've also taken in the benefit of dealing with oneself, care, and self-compassion.

Realising that you have the stuff to plan the existence you need, I believe you should feel more engaged and brimming with conceivable outcomes when you put this book down. I want to believe that you will respect your body, psyche, and soul in each choice you make and embrace every day with veritable reason. Additionally, may you find contentment and happiness while travelling, embracing the challenges, and applauding your accomplishments.

You have tremendous potential and are ready to do significantly more than you comprehend. Keep your own solidarity in mind; have faith in both your objectives and yourself. As you start your excursion of self-revelation and self-awareness, may you generally dare to pay attention to your instinct and the insight to pay attention to your inward voice.

I am very grateful to you for allowing me to be a part of your experience. May you have

Learner Stronger energy

many opportunities, love, and light. Cheers to your flourishing, charm, and endless possible results! The world is keeping it together for the amazing splendour of your soul, so go out and thrive.

With thanks and appreciation,

[Rosendo A. Price]